FOOD TO EAT BEFORE AND AFTER SEX

Foods you should eat before and after sex to gain energy.

Dr. Henry C. Law

Table of contents

Chapter 1

EAT THIS BEFORE AND AFTER SEX:

Dark chocolate

While the evidence is still out on whether or not aphrodisiacs truly function as advertised, this typical alternative is nonetheless ideal to consume before sex for a few simple reasons:

Dark chocolate is chock-full of anandamide and phenylethylamine (PEA), which is regarded as the love chemical.
Both chemicals improve your mood by releasing happy hormones (also known as endorphins).

Phenylethylamine is also important for controlling physical energy and attention and is connected to a sensation of emotional bliss, boosting blood pressure and heart rate.

Sounds a lot like sex, doesn't it? However, owing to another element, methylxanthines, the energy advantages are sadly short-lived, so don't consume it too much ahead of a possible sexy time.

In addition, a recent 2021 study also discovered that chocolate may not only excite but also emulate sex closely for certain women, actually diminishing their desire for sex since researchers theorized it might duplicate it in our brains.

Avocados

To offset the generally short-lived effects of chocolate, try avocados. This green fruit is one of those nutritious kitchen mainstays that maintain your energy for the long haul, and its relationship to sexual function isn't a new one; in fact, the name stems from the Nahuatl (language of the Aztecs) and means "testicle."

(Yes, you read it properly.) Avocados are high in monounsaturated (good) fats, minerals, and vitamin B6 (essential for maintaining our energy and sexual drive), according to experts.Not to mention that avocados are great for your overall health and can help keep your skin and other organs healthy.

Strawberries

While we're on avocados, let's also examine the following fruity choices to get you in the mood: This fruit salad of good-for-you foods is also oh-so-good for your sexual life. Strawberries are not just a sexy-looking fruit (our eyes are naturally attracted to red), but they're chock-full of zinc, antioxidants, and vitamin C, which enhances libido.

Zinc is vital to sexual health and plays a role in both testosterone management (what sperm creation relies on) and vaginal lubrication, which prepares the female form for sex. It's really the strawberry seeds that contain the zinc, and although we don't consume the seeds in most fruits, strawberries are the exception here.

Watermelon

While watermelon is very hydrating and obviously tasty to eat before sex, its prior association with having "natural Viagra-like effects" was actually refuted by McGill University. Still, it's not to suggest that it isn't an excellent go-to for pre-sex. Watermelon includes citrulline, which is a renowned mood booster, like chocolate.

Apples

This simple snack is a fast way to refresh your breath and eliminate any food particles from your teeth. If you're wondering which additional fruits to include in your "sex fruit salad," bananas, pomegranate seeds, and figs are also wonderful for your sexual wellbeing and drive in the boudoir.

Nuts

Obvious jokes aside, like strawberry seeds, nuts (think: cashews and almonds) are filled with zinc, which touts sexual advantages. Additionally, one 2019 study indicated that incorporating nuts into a regular diet increased orgasmic performance and sexual drive in guys. Now we only need to study how food affects women's sexual health.

Crushed flax seeds

Seeds (like nuts) are good foods to consume for your sexual health, and they too are rich providers of zinc. Flax seeds are a recognized superfood, rich in antioxidants, and related to improving blood flow to your sexy parts.

The omega-3s are fantastic for your cardiovascular health, which plays a part in your libido. Amino acids may help enhance blood flow and keep sperm healthy. Additionally, experts claim that flax seeds may even have a moderating influence on hormones in menopausal women.

Chia seeds

These little seeds are nutritious powerhouses in disguise. They carry a ton of energy to keep you going (and lasting) long into the night (or day).

Pumpkin seeds

They, like flax seeds, contain a high concentration of Omega-3 fatty acids, which are beneficial to both gynecological and prostate health (roasted pumpkin seeds have even been linked to improving erectile function in male rats in one study).Additionally, they are full of iron, which helps us feel stimulated, and magnesium, which helps us feel calm.

Ginger

Not only can ginger freshen breath, but it has been proven to promote circulation and widen the blood vessels, which improves blood flow to the genitals and, in turn, stimulates desire.

AVOID THESE MEALS BEFORE HAVING SEX:

Bad news for charcuterie boards everywhere: as a general rule, it's preferable to avoid highly-processed, salty, and fatty meals, which may trigger cramps and flatulence. Here are a few additional items you should skip.

Imagine you went out with a gorgeous date, and after a romantic meal, you're in need of some exercise—happens to all of us, doesn't it? But immediately then, your stomach displays its disapproval: you feel excessively bloated, and your desire diminishes too! You may wonder what occurred all of a sudden, but it's the food you ate at supper playing spoilsport.

We all know the sorts of foods that may put the heat up in the bedroom, but how about those that kill the vibe?

That's why we are here to educate you about all the meals you must avoid if you're searching for some sexy time with your date.

Avoid this before sex:

Cheese

While cheese might be a delightful finger food to nibble on, it's dairy and, as such, can function as a congestant and mucous-builder for many individuals (not to mention bloating), leading many to not feel their best going into a sex session. Additionally, if the dairy originates from cow's milk, it might contain hormones that interfere with our biological processes.

Beans

This may be an apparent one, but there's a reason Bart Simpson sang about beans being the musical fruit... It boils down to beans having high quantities of raffinose, a kind of carbohydrate that's poorly processed by the body. Needless to say, gassiness doesn't make anybody feel sexy, even though the bean is a terrific plant-based meat replacement. Maybe just avoid it before exercising.

Too much red wine or other alcohol

While a glass (or two) may certainly reduce inhibitions and provide some liquid confidence, drinking too much can make us tired (before eventually upsetting our deep rest) (before eventually disrupting our deep slumber).However, for males too, drinking too much might damage male sexual function.

black licorice

ItIt may seem like a weird addition to this list, but black licorice has been associated withwith reducingreducing testosterone levels,levels, and testosterone is significantly connected to sex desire in both men and women.

chips

Foods like chips that are heavy in saturated (bad) fats aren't great for your love life. This is because over time they may harm your circulation, impede blood flow,flow, and impair your sexualsexual organ performance. Think of it as undoing all the hard work of all those good-for-your-circulation meals we described before.

Spicy food

If you want to spice up your sex life, then it's time to avoid spicy meals before intercourse. Spicy food might induce acid reflux, indigestion,indigestion, or even prompt you to go to the bathroom a thousand times, not something you'd want, isn't it?

Onions with garlic

We all know how onions and garlic can give us bad breath, but that's not all, they may also affect the scent of your secretions.Yes, it's true. Pungent foods are a major no-no before sex, so simply stay away from caramelizedcaramelized onions or your favoritefavorite garlic chutney before the big night!

Desserts

If sweet snacks make you weak in the knees, then there's some terrible news for you. All those sugar-laden cakes and sweets might damage your sexualsexual pleasure. That's because sweets are filled with trans fat and sugar and might hinder you from reaching the big O.

That's not all;; the sweetness also boosts the insulin levels in your body, and that's not what you want in the bedroom.

Starchy carbohydrates

We all know junk food equals an abundance of carbohydrates, but ingesting too much might drop your blood sugar levels, and that'll make you very lethargic! If you want to spice up your sexualsexual life, forgo any carb-heavy meal like fries, rice,rice, or pasta pasta.

Soy products

Soy might be healthy, but consuming excessive amounts can cause hormonal imbalance, and that means low libido! So, if you're a vegan, avoid soy before a hot and heavy session in the bedroom.

Carbonated drinks

It's a no-brainer that carbonated beverages are bad, but guess what?? TheyThey are the worst beverage to consume before sex! That's because it may make you bloated and gassy. You don't want your lovemaking session to be interrupted by farts and burps! Gross, isn't it?

Salty food

Last but not least, avoid salty meals before sex! That's because meals filled with salt make you feel bloated in no time. Apart from that, it might also hinder you from attaining an orgasm by lowering your blood flow. You certainly don't want that, right?

So, women, the next time you're out on a romantic date, skip these meals and have hot sex like never before.

Chapter 2

CHANGES IN THE BODY

Here are ways in which your body changes when you start having sex.

When you start having sex, you will feel quite a few changes in your body. Here are some of them.

If you have recently begun having sex, you will feel quite a few changes in your body. We know you have a lot of questions regarding what will be different from now on. While these changes range from person to person, here's a list of changes you are likely to encounter:

1. You could be in pain.

Painful sex is a genuine phenomenon, and there might be a range of different causes for it.

However, the explanations are really fairly frequent and nothing to be frightened about. You might be feeling discomfort due to your hymen being stretched. It might be because of a lack of lubrication due to vaginal dryness.

This might occur owing to a disorder called vaginismus, which is an involuntary tightening of the pelvic muscles that makes it hard for anything to enter the vagina. It has a normal relationship with anxiety, which stems from a rigid and religious upbringing, trauma baggage, or simply plain fear.

Sometimes, if you have previously orgasmed during sex, it might cause you to have cramping in your uterus. It is the oxytocin release in the body that produces uterine contractions and, consequently, the discomfort.

2. There could be sightings.

You could bleed after intercourse, but you also might not. Either way, it is completely fine. You could bleed when you have penetrative intercourse for the first time, and that might be due to your hymen breaking. The hymen is a tiny patch of skin protecting the opening of the vagina.

It breaks pretty readily, and sex doesn't have to be the primary reason why it breaks. It might break due to severe physical activity, such as horseback riding and other sports, or even from wearing tampons. A damaged hymen doesn't always indicate that your virginity is gone.

Apart from that, if you detect a tiny amount of spotting, it might be due to the inflammation of the cervix that becomes constricted during sex or owing to vaginal tearing if you are having hard sex. The blood flowing from an irritated cervix or vaginal tears is generally bright crimson. If it's darker in color, it is usually remnant blood from your periods.

3. You could experience a burning feeling.

It's alright if you feel a burn when you make a trip to the bathroom post-sex. The urethra and the vagina are closely situated. The vaginal strain or tear might be creating a brief burning sensation. However, if you have this ache for days, it might be something dangerous.

4. You can have itching.

If you are bothered by the impulse to scratch an itch after sex, you are probably allergic or sensitive to the condom that you used. It might also be sensitive to lubrication if you have used some.

5. You can acquire a urinary tract infection.

In the process of having sex, a transfer of germs from the gut to the vaginal canal and up to the urethra may happen. This might be the source of a severe UTI that can produce itching and a burning feeling.

6. The size of your nipples and clitoris can shift.

Your nipples are loaded with nerve endings, which become revved up when you are aroused. They cause the blood vessels to dilate and the tissue in your breasts to swell up. This sexual excitement also leads to erections in your nipples.

Similarly, if you start having sex, you will have your clitoris swell up throughout the deed. It will, however, return to its regular size after a few minutes. This occurs due to increased blood flow in the pelvic area.

7. You'll feel the surge of happy hormones.

Once you start having sex, your body begins feeling increased blood flow and muscle tension in locations like your nipples, areola, and clitoris. Upon being aroused, you experience goosebumps, your areola expands, and the nipples get firm. All of these contribute to your orgasm, all because of the oxytocin release occurring in your brain.

8. Your vaginal elasticity will alter

Your vagina understands how to modify its suppleness. The walls and lips of your vagina gently open up during arousal. Don’t worry, your vagina is designed to grow and prepare you for sex.

So, ladies, now that you’re more aware of everything that is going to happen to your body when you start having sex.

Chapter 3

SEXUAL HEALTH

We hired a gynecologist to address all your concerns regarding having sex after pregnancy.

Too many questions swirling in your brain about having sex after pregnancy? Worry not; we've got all the answers for you.

If you thought nine months of pregnancy was the ultimate roller coaster journey of emotions, prepare yourself for more! Most first-time moms are unaware that the body goes through a lot of changes once the child is born. And just as it isn't simple to snap back to your prior lifestyle after delivery, it will also take some time to experience enjoyable sex after pregnancy.

We know you have loads of hot concerns on this issue, which is why we've asked Dr. Sandeep Chadha, consultant obstetrician and gynecologist at the Motherhood Hospital, Noida, to answer them all for you!

How soon can you have sex after childbirth?

Whether you've experienced a C-section or regular delivery, Dr. Chadha recommended you wait for six weeks before engaging in sexual intercourse. After all, your body needs time to recuperate after birth! He also suggests contacting a gynecologist to confirm that the incision is healing nicely and that postpartum bleeding has ceased.

"Following the birth, your body enters a healing period when the bleeding ceases, the rips mend, and the cervix shuts. "Having intercourse too early, particularly during the first 2 weeks, increases the risk of postpartum hemorrhage or uterine infection," says Dr. Chadha.

Pregnancy may be daunting. So allow your body the time it needs.

What changes might you anticipate in your sexual life?

-

You may believe post-pregnancy means zero sex, but that's absolutely not true! Just that, it may take some time to spice things up in the bedroom.Until then, it's essential to be psychologically prepared and cope with the following changes:

1. Your breasts will feel delicate, which may cause pain during intercourse.

2. After a normal birth, your vagina splits off and requires time to mend. Don't become disappointed, but sex could not feel the way it did before the birth of your kid.

3. You could suffer from body image problems and feel ugly owing to severe postpartum stress and weight gain.

4. If this is your first pregnancy, you could feel much more weary and fatigued during intercourse.

While these anxieties make you feel down and out, don't forget to be proud of yourself for bringing a kid into this world!

What should you do to guarantee a healthy and enjoyable sexual life?

While sex after pregnancy is different, it doesn't have to be horrible. Dr. Chadha advises, "Have an open talk with your spouse about what makes you feel good and what doesn't. This can help you enjoy sex again and make sure you are not feeling any unnecessary pain.

Here's everything that you can do:

1. Take it slow:

In the first few weeks post-delivery, your body may not be ready for all that heated activity.

Give yourself some time and space, and take things one day at a time.

2. Engage in more foreplay.

Allow your vagina to develop its own natural lubrication before the intercourse.Longer foreplay implies less pain.

3. Don't hesitate to use lubes:

You could need some aid with lubrication since your hormones are still out of line. While buying lubes, go for a water-based choice, as the oil-based ones might break condoms and irritate your delicate tissue.

4. Make Kegel exercises your best friend.

Kegel exercises may be quite useful, particularly during the postpartum recovery period. It helps to restore pelvic floor muscles and may assist in easing post-delivery disorders, including urinary incontinence. All in all, these exercises will aid in recovering power and sensitivity in the vagina, making sex more delightful!

Contrary to what you may believe, having kids does not imply zero sex. Slowly and slowly, things will heat up in the bedroom again—it's just a matter of time.

Chapter 4

WHAT TO DRINK AFTER SEX

Should We Drink Water Just After Sex?

There have been speculations and rumors about the risks of drinking water after intercourse. From a medical viewpoint, how much truth is there?

There are no clear solutions to this subject of whether we should drink water right after sex, nor is there any research that reveals any possible concerns related to drinking water after sex.

However, the preponderance of data shows that drinking water before, during, or after intercourse is crucial because:

Sexual activity drains strength, so it is essential to keep drinking water after sex to hydrate and maintain energy levels.

Drinking a glass of water after sex improves sexual hygiene by enhancing the production of pee. This, in turn, helps eliminate unwanted germs from the body and prevents infections.

It's necessary to flush out toxins from the body, which may be done with greater water intake.

Drinking enough water keeps the penis well-supplied with blood and oxygen.

benefits of drinking water after sex

There are various advantages to drinking water after intercourse, some of which are described below:

1. Increased lubrication

Have a problem with dryness in your lower body? Start increasing the quantity of water you consume since dehydration may cause dryness in the private areas, resulting in uncomfortable sex.

2. Improved Orgasms

Not only are you more lubricated when you're hydrated, but there's also increased blood flow to your penis, resulting in better and longer orgasms.

3. Increases Your Energy Levels

Appropriate water consumption can help you feel more energized. Poor hydration impacts the energy-generating processes in the body, leaving you with poor endurance and energy for sex.

4. It Cleanses Your Vital System

Water washes toxins and impurities out of your body naturally. All of these substances may build up in your tissues if you don't drink enough water, disrupting your body's delicate biochemical equilibrium. This will subsequently affect your libido and sex hormones, making you less eager for sex.

5. It alleviates weariness.

A powerful sex session may be as tiring as exercise. According to recent research, 25 to 30 minutes of sexual activity is similar to a 3-mile run. There is also a post-sex energy dip. Water could aid you in fighting the tiredness that comes with sexual activity.

Drinking water alone after sexual intercourse may not be adequate; sexual intercourse is perceived as a strenuous physical activity, which it may frequently be.

1. Electrolyte water

If you sweat abundantly during sex, you may be losing electrolytes, which must be replaced as the human body demands them.

2. Coconut Water

High in magnesium, salt, potassium, and vitamin C, coconut water is good for drinking after sex. These nutrients are not present in regular water.

3. Banana Shake

One of the side effects of sex is cramping. So, drinking a banana shake after sex helps prevent muscle spasms or cramps. Bananas, according to nutritionists, contain the enzyme bromelain, which has been shown in some studies to increase a man's libido.

They're also high in B vitamins like riboflavin, which are necessary for producing testosterone, the sex hormone.

4. Buttermilk

Buttermilk is produced from yoghurt, which includes calcium, vitamins B6 and B12, riboflavin, potassium, and magnesium. These critical nutrients assist in maintaining healthy balance and energy in the body after sex.

5. Cranberry juice

Cranberry juice is among the most commonly suggested natural beverages to boost urine output in the body, via which toxins may be flushed out.

Chapter 5

UNPROTECTED SEX

This Is What You Should Do If You Have Unprotected Sex or If Your Condom Fails.

If you've had sex without a condom or a sexual encounter when the condom broke, try not to worry.

Things happen, and you're far from the first person to go through any of these situations.

What you do need to understand, however, is that there are a few hazards involved with these sexual activities.

But there are lots of things you can do to address those dangers so that you stay safe and sexually healthy.

Immediately after:

If you notice that the condom has broken, stop all sexual activity and leave your partner.

If you've had sex without a condom, remember that there are a few things you can do immediately to help.

Use the bathroom:

First, travel to the restroom to remove residual secretions from the vagina, penis, or anus.

This may make you feel more comfortable and help eliminate germs that might result in urinary tract infections (UTIs).

You may sit on the toilet and press down with your genital or anal muscles to expel any residual fluid. Peeing might also help.

Just know that if you have a vulva and have had penis-in-vagina intercourse, peeing won't decrease the possibility of pregnancy. That's because the sperm has already moved toward the egg.

Don't douche, but do wash up.

It's a fallacy that genital parts require thorough cleansing after sexual activity.

While cleaning and drying genital regions might further boost your comfort, vaginal or anal douching can actually put you at higher risk of an infection.

This is because douching products may cause irritation and inflammation.

So if you wish to wash, just take a shower or use tepid water to sprinkle the area.

Check in with yourself.

Make sure you take time to ask yourself how you're feeling.

It's common to feel a broad variety of emotions following intercourse without a condom, whether that's concern, rage, or despair.

Try to talk to friends or relatives about the problem so that they can assist you.

If you aren't comfortable speaking to anybody you know, try reaching out to Planned Parenthood or the National Coalition for Sexual Health for support.

Plan out your next steps.

Once you're feeling more comfortable, it's a good idea to think about what to do next.

If you require emergency contraception (EC), take a look at where your local drugstore is and its operating hours. Some types of EC are available over-the-counter and don't need a doctor's prescription.

If you're afraid that you may have been exposed to a sexually transmitted infection

(STI) or HIV, arrange an appointment with a doctor or sexual health clinic.

Remember that you only need to have oral or penetrative intercourse with someone once to develop an STI.

Watch for symptoms:

While some STIs might be symptomless, others may show up in the form of sores, itching, foul discharge, or discomfort while peeing.

Keep an eye on your genitals, anus, and mouth region and arrange an STI test if you see anything strange.

Within 3 days:

Some kinds of EC need to be taken within 72 hours after intercourse without a condom.

Similarly, it's crucial to take prophylactic medicine for HIV during the same period.

Get PEP from a healthcare professional:

If you're afraid that you may have caught HIV, post-exposure prophylaxis (PEP) can minimize your chance of obtaining an infection.

Starting the therapy as soon as feasible, preferably within a few hours after probable exposure, is critical to its efficacy.

You'll need to take it once or twice a day for at least 28 days, and it may not be successful for everyone.

When it does work, the combination of pills—known as antiretroviral medications—stops HIV from multiplying and spreading throughout the body.

Get Plan B or another levonorgestrel EC tablet from your local pharmacy:

EC tablets aim to prevent conception by suppressing biological processes like ovulation.

EC tablets containing a synthetic hormone called levonorgestrel need to be taken within 72 hours after intercourse for optimal efficacy.

Talk with a healthcare expert about ella or ParaGard.

Other forms of EC exist to assist in preventing pregnancy.

These include ella, a pill that may be taken up to 5 days after intercourse, and ParaGard, an intrauterine device (IUD) that can be used as a long-term birth control technique.

To access any of these choices, you'll need to consult a doctor.

Within 5 days:

While over-the-counter forms of EC should be taken within 3 days after intercourse or condom rupture for the greatest chance of avoiding pregnancy, prescription techniques are safer to use within 5 days.

If you haven't used EC yet, Ela and ParaGard are equally effective until day 5:

ParaGard is the most successful type of EC, with just 1 in 1,000 individuals falling pregnant following usage.

It also works just as effectively on day 5 as it did on day 1, so you don't have to worry so much about time.

Of course, it will need a doctor's visit and a sometimes pricey charge.

But since the copper makes it difficult for sperm to reach an egg, it may be used as regular birth control for up to a decade.

Another alternative is Ella.

It stops or delays ovulation by suppressing the hormone progesterone and decreases pregnancy chances by 85 percent if taken within 5 days after intercourse.

Plan B and other levonorgestrel tablets are less effective but may still be used:

If you've gone over the 72-hour limit, you may still take a levonorgestrel EC pill, including Plan B, for another 2 days.

But the longer you wait to take it, the less effective it is at reducing the probability of pregnancy.

2 weeks later:

Unusual discharge and discomfort while peeing are frequent signs of both gonorrhea and chlamydia.

You should also watch out for bleeding after intercourse and between cycles.

Pain might also arise in the throat.

trusted source if gonorrhea arises through oral intercourse and in the stomach or testicles as a consequence of chlamydia.

However, other individuals may have no symptoms at all.

So it's crucial to obtain a test for both of these STIs 2 weeks after intercourse, since they may lead to more significant difficulties, such as infertility.

Waiting roughly 14 days following possible exposure is regarded as the interval that delivers the most accurate findings.

Trusted Source.

If you obtain a positive test, remember that both STIs are curable with medication, and you should avoid having intercourse until the illness clears.

3 weeks later:

If you're afraid you could be pregnant, the first indicator tends to be a missing period.

You'll need to take a pregnancy test to find out for sure.

Pregnancy tests operate by detecting a hormone called human chorionic gonadotropin (hCG). It might take a long time for enough hCG to build up in your body; therefore, you should wait to take a test until 3 weeks after intercourse.

If the test is positive, arrange an appointment with a healthcare expert to explore your choices.

When it comes to testing for genital herpes and HIV, realize that there isn't a treatment for either of these illnesses.

You may recognize genital herpes as blisters that leave open sores or as a burning or itchy feeling.

HIV may mimic the flu. But once these short-term symptoms fade, you may not notice anything unusual.

Waiting at least 3 weeks to get tested for HIV and genital herpes is required, since both have a fairly long incubation period. This implies you may have a false negative if you get tested too soon.

Although the viruses will always stay in your body, there are therapies available.

Antiviral medication may improve genital herpes symptoms if required. Similar sorts of treatment may also stop HIV from multiplying.

6 weeks later:

Syphilis is another STI that may be hard to recognize; in fact, you may have no symptoms at all.

However, it's crucial to be checked since it might create long-term health issues in numerous sections of the body.

-

Signs of syphilis that may occur include:

- tiny blisters or growths in your genital region or mouth.
- blotchy rash on the palms of hands or soles of feet
- fever
- headaches
- joint discomfort

The incubation period might be much longer than other illnesses; therefore, wait roughly 6 weeks to get tested for a more trustworthy result.

If it's positive, you'll be prescribed a course of antibiotics. Again, avoid any sexual activity until the illness has entirely resolved.

3 months later:

It's usually a good idea to test for any of the aforementioned STIs again a few months after intercourse without a condom or condom failure.

This might help you feel confident that any negative result you obtained is actually negative and that whatever therapy you received has worked.

When it comes to syphilis, in particular, it's advisable to undergo retests after 3 and 6 months.

This will monitor for recurring infections and confirm that treatment has been effective, particularly since syphilis has shown evidence of antibiotic resistance.

Trusted Source.

Things to consider for next time:

Accidents happen, and, in rare situations, you may actively choose to have sex without a condom.

If you're at all concerned about the possible implications, prepare yourself by contemplating the following:

Barrier methods:

Using a barrier approach, you can reduce your chances of getting an STI.

This comprises condoms, gloves, and dental dams for oral sex.

When using condoms, verify that they aren't expired, and avoid opening the container with sharp items to prevent inadvertent nicks or wounds on the surface.

Secondary contraception:

While condoms can help prevent STIs, they may present certain complications if used as contraception.

If you want a more dependable technique, think about taking an extra type of birth control, whether it's a pill or a more long-term option like an IUD.

Regular STI screening:

Getting tested for STIs on a regular basis is crucial for your sexual health. You may arrange a test with a healthcare practitioner or via a sexual health center.

It's good to be tested at least once a year. If you have several relationships, try boosting this trusted source every 3 to 6 months.

Remember to be honest and upfront with your relationships, too.

The bottom line:

Whether you've consciously had sex without a condom or suffered an accident with a condom, there are lots of actions you can take to care for your sexual health and prevent pregnancy.

Keeping oneself safe on an ongoing basis is easy, too. All you need is a barrier approach and dependable contraception.

www.ingramcontent.com/pod-product-compliance
Lightning Source LLC
LaVergne TN
LVHW020524160826
845677LV00015B/3884

* 9 7 9 8 3 6 6 4 7 4 0 6 1 *